THE TELL ALL GUIDE TO BEAT CANCER

Take Control of Your Health and Fight Cancer!

By: PETER E.STEVENSON

Introduction

The sun shone brightly through the window, warming the room with its beaming light. It was a day like any other, yet something felt different. On this particular morning, 18-year-old Sarah awoke with a strange feeling of unease in her stomach. She had no idea what was causing it, but the feeling was unmistakable.

Little did she know that on that very morning, her entire life would change. Later that day, Sarah went in for a routine physical at the doctor's office. After a few tests, the doctor's face grew pale. He informed Sarah that she had cancer.

Suddenly, Sarah's world was spinning out of control. She had never expected something like this to happen to her. She had always been healthy and happy. How could this be happening?

The next few months were a blur of hospital visits and treatments. Sarah was in and out of doctor's offices and hospitals, trying her best to fight against the disease. But, it seemed no matter how hard she tried, it was slowly but surely taking over her body.

Through it all, Sarah was surrounded by family and friends who provided her with love, support, and encouragement. They helped her to stay positive and look to the future. Though it wasn't easy, Sarah was determined to beat the cancer and be healthy again.

After months of treatments and hospital visits, Sarah was finally cancer-free. She was able to return to her normal life and start living her life again. Though she had been through so much, she was determined to make the most of her second chance.

Sarah was able to look back on her experience with cancer with a newfound appreciation for life. She was determined to live each day to the fullest, cherishing each moment and never taking a single breath for granted. She was grateful for all that she had been through and the lessons she had learned along the way.

Cancer may have been a devastating experience, but it was also a life-changing one. Through it all, Sarah was able to find strength and courage to keep fighting and never lose hope. Her story is a reminder of the power of the human spirit and an inspiration to all those facing similar struggles.

Sarah's cancer story is a heartwarming reminder of the resilience of the human spirit and the power of hope in the face of adversity. She is a shining example of the power of courage and determination to overcome any obstacle. Through her experience, she was able to find strength in the darkest of times and a newfound appreciation for life.

Her story is a reminder that no matter how dark the night, the sun will always rise again.

sarah was able to beat cancer and find a new appreciation for life. Through her experience, she was able to find strength and courage to keep fighting and never lose hope. Her story is a reminder of the power of the human spirit and an inspiration to all those facing similar struggles. Cancer may have been a devastating experience, but it is also a story of hope and courage that will continue to inspire for years to come.

Cancer is a devastating disease that affects millions of people every year. It is a complex condition that can have many different causes and treatments. It is estimated that over 1.7

million new cases of cancer are diagnosed each year in the United States alone, with a projected 14.5 million new cases worldwide in 2020. Cancer is the second leading cause of death in the United States after heart disease.

Cancer is a disease caused by changes to the genetic material of cells. These changes can cause cells to divide and grow uncontrollably, forming malignant tumors. Cancer cells can spread to other organs, forming secondary tumors. This process is known as metastasis.

Cancer can affect almost any part of the body, including organs, blood, and lymphatic systems. It is classified into four main types: carcinoma, sarcoma, leukemia, and lymphoma. Carcinomas are malignancies that originate in the skin, lining of organs and glands, or connective tissue. Sarcomas start in the body's connective tissue, such as muscle, cartilage, fat, and bone. Leukemia is a cancer of the blood, and lymphoma is a cancer of the lymphatic system.

The causes of cancer are still not fully understood, but some factors are known to increase the risk. These include age, genetics, lifestyle, and environmental factors. Smoking, excessive alcohol consumption, and radiation exposure have been linked to an increased risk of certain types of cancer.

Treatments for cancer vary depending on the type and stage of the disease. Surgery, chemotherapy, radiation therapy, and immunotherapy are all common treatments.

Cancer is a complex and difficult disease to face. However, advances in diagnosis and treatments have made it much more manageable. With early diagnosis and appropriate treatment, cancer can often be successfully managed or even cured. It is important to understand your risk factors, get regular check-ups, and seek medical help when needed.

No matter how daunting the battle against cancer may be, there is help and hope. Cancer research is ongoing, and new treatments are being developed every day. Support and resources are available to those affected by the disease, and there is strength in knowing that you are not alone.

CHAPTER ONE

MY LIFE BEFORE

My life before cancer was filled with adventure and exploration. I was an active and determined individual who enjoyed the outdoors and taking risks. I loved to challenge myself and was always looking for ways to push my physical and mental boundaries. I was an avid traveler and had the privilege of visiting a variety of countries around the world. I had the opportunity to experience different cultures and traditions, as well as different lifestyles. I was exposed to different ideas, perspectives, and beliefs that changed the way I thought and acted. I also had a great career. I enjoyed my job as an accountant and I was passionate about helping people. I was constantly learning new skills and expanding my knowledge base. In addition to my career, I had a number of hobbies that I enjoyed, such as cooking and reading. I had a large network of friends and family who I shared many special moments with, and I made sure to make time for myself to relax and enjoy life. Above all, I was truly enjoying life and everything that came with it. I had a strong sense of self and felt like I was making a difference in the world. I was filled with energy and optimism and had a positive outlook on the future. Unfortunately, all of this changed when I was diagnosed with cancer. I was suddenly thrust into a world of uncertainty and fear. I was scared and confused and felt like my life was spinning out of control. While this experience was undoubtedly difficult, it also taught me a lot about myself. I learned how to be resilient, how to take things one day at a time, and how to appreciate the small moments in life. Now, I am in remission and living life to the fullest. I am grateful for the life I have and all the lessons I have learned along the way. I am determined to continue pushing my boundaries and reminding myself to appreciate every moment. No matter what life throws at me, I know I have the strength and courage to face it head on. being diagnosed with cancer didn't stop me. It only made me stronger. don't let cancer defeat you, let it motivate you.

Living with a diagnosis of any kind can be a difficult and challenging process. It can be especially daunting if the diagnosis comes suddenly, as mine did. After being diagnosed with a chronic illness, I was faced with a lot of fear and uncertainty about my future. I was scared of the unknown, and filled with questions about how my life would be different.

But I quickly realized that I was the only one who could take control of my situation and decide how to live my life after diagnosis. With that realization, I made a commitment to myself to live my life to the fullest, despite any challenges or limitations I faced.

The first step I took was to learn as much as I could about my condition. I read books, attended seminars, and talked to other people with a similar diagnosis. I got to know my body better, and learned what I could do to stay as healthy and active as possible.

Once I had a better understanding of my situation, I made lifestyle changes to accommodate my diagnosis. I began to practice regular self-care, including eating healthier, getting more sleep, and exercising regularly. I also made an effort to become more organized and efficient with my time.

I also decided that it was important to stay connected with my friends and family. I was worried that my diagnosis would make it hard for me to be a part of their lives, but I chose to reach out anyway. I kept in touch through phone calls, video chats, and messages. I also made sure to attend special events and gatherings, even if I had to rest or take breaks throughout.

I also took up new activities and hobbies that I enjoyed, such as painting, writing, and cooking. These activities provided me with a sense of purpose and accomplishment. I also used my experiences to help others by volunteering and speaking at community events.

Finally, I made sure to take time for myself to relax and recharge. I practiced mindfulness and meditation, took long walks, and spent time in nature. I also made sure to take regular vacations, both near and far, so I could escape the stress of my day-to-day life.

Living with a diagnosis can be a difficult and challenging experience, but it doesn't have to be debilitating. I have found that by taking control of my situation and making positive lifestyle changes, I can still live a fulfilling life. I have come to appreciate the little moments and treasured memories that I make each day. We all have challenges in life, but we can choose how we respond to them. I chose to take the path of resilience, and I am so glad I did.

CHAPTER TWO

CANCER SYMPTOMS AND ANNOUNCEMENT OF MY CANCER

It was a day like any other when I got the news that changed my life. I was diagnosed with cancer. I was in shock and disbelief, not knowing how to process the news that I was facing a life-threatening illness. I was scared and unsure of what the future would bring.

My doctor had informed me that I had a tumor in my abdomen and I needed to begin treatment immediately. I felt overwhelmed and scared by the thought of going through treatments and the potential side effects. I had so many questions about my prognosis and what the future would bring.

I took some time to process the news and think about how I wanted to handle this situation. I knew that I wanted to be proactive and take control of my health. I decided that I wanted to be open and honest with my loved ones and share my diagnosis.

I took to social media to share the news that I had cancer. I wrote a post on my Facebook page and shared it with my friends and family. I was open and honest about my diagnosis and what I was going through. I shared with them that I was scared but determined to fight this disease and beat it.

I was overwhelmed by the outpouring of love and support that I received from my family and friends. They all offered kind words of encouragement, prayers, and support. I felt so blessed to have such wonderful people in my life.

I also shared my story with the media. I wanted to raise awareness about my diagnosis, and to inspire people who were facing similar challenges. I wanted to show them that, even in the face of adversity, you can still be strong and fight for your health.

I am now a few months into my treatment and I am grateful for the progress that I have made. My cancer is still a challenge, but I am determined to keep fighting and beating it. I want to raise awareness about cancer, and to show people that no matter how difficult the journey may be, they can still find strength and hope.

I am so thankful for the support that I have received from my family, friends, and strangers who have been inspired by my story. I hope that by sharing my experience, I can help inspire others to fight for their health, no matter how difficult the journey may be.

there is relief in informing your loved ones about your diagnosis. That's why I chose to be open and honest with my diagnosis and share it with my friends and family. I wanted to give them the opportunity to provide me with the support I need. I hope that my story will help others going through a similar situation and show them that, even in the face of adversity, you can still be strong and fight for your health.

my family gave me all the support I need in battling cancer. I am so thankful for their love and support throughout this difficult time.

I believe that it is important to share your story and be open and honest about your diagnosis. By doing this, you can help raise awareness about cancer and inspire others who are struggling with similar issues.

CHAPTER THREE

MY DETERMINATION TO FIGHT FOR SURVIVAL

As humans, we are blessed with the ability to adapt, learn, and ultimately survive. I have experienced this firsthand through my own determination to fight for survival.

Growing up in an impoverished family in a developing country, I have seen firsthand the struggles of making ends meet. When I was younger, I didn't understand the importance of money and the struggles my parents faced to keep food on the table. I was too young to comprehend the difficulty of sustaining a family with limited resources.

However, I soon began to comprehend the gravity of the situation when my parents could no longer afford to pay for my school fees. I was forced to drop out of school and start working to provide for my family. This experience was a turning point in my life and it was then that I realized the importance of money and the need to fight for survival.

I started working in a small shop and eventually worked my way up to managing it. With the little money I earned, I started investing in small businesses and eventually saved enough to open my own shop. This was a huge milestone for me and it gave me the confidence to keep fighting for survival.

In the years that followed, I continued to grow my business, eventually becoming quite successful. I started to understand the importance of hard work and the power of determination. With a bit of luck and a lot of hard work, I was able to provide a better life for my family.

My story is a testament to the power of determination and the importance of survival. I have seen firsthand the power of perseverance and the ability to turn a difficult situation into an opportunity. No matter the odds, I have always been determined to fight for survival and use my experiences to inspire others.

The world can be a harsh place, but with a bit of determination, anything is possible. I believe that no matter what life throws at you, it is possible to fight for survival and create a better future. With a bit of hard work and determination, anything is possible.

my determination kept me going and it is what drives me to this day.

if you're willing to fight against cancer, poverty, or even just the odds, you can make it. That's what I believe in.

Cancer can be overwhelming sometimes but determination to fight it has saved many lives. It's not only the medical treatments that save lives, it's the determination to fight.

No matter the odds, I believe that it is possible to fight for survival and create a better future. With a bit of hard work and determination, anything is possible. That is what I have learned from my own experiences and that is what I continue to believe in. With a bit of determination and hard work, anything is possible.

CHAPTER FOUR

My next life

Living with cancer is a harrowing experience that no one should ever have to go through. It is a life-altering journey and a rollercoaster of emotions that can be overwhelming to process. It is a journey of hope and courage, and it is one that no one should have to go through alone.

For those living with cancer, it is important to remember that you are not alone. There are thousands of others just like you, who are going through similar struggles and experiences. By connecting with these individuals, you can not only provide support for one another, but also gain strength and hope for the future.

It is also important to focus on the positive aspects of life and to stay positive. This can be done by engaging in activities that bring you happiness, such as reading, listening to music, or spending time with family and friends. Doing these things can help you to refocus your energy and put things into perspective.

It is also important to take care of yourself and to find ways to manage your stress. This can include talking to a therapist or joining a support group. Meditation, yoga, and regular exercise can also be beneficial.

Seeking out medical treatments and therapies can also help to manage the symptoms of your cancer. This can include chemotherapy, radiation, and other specialized treatments. It is important to talk to your doctor about the best treatment plan for your specific situation and to stay informed on the latest developments in cancer treatment.

It is also important to remember that living with cancer can be unpredictable. There will be days when you are feeling strong and optimistic, and other days when you feel discouraged and overwhelmed. It is important to recognize and accept these feelings, as they are a natural part of the process.

Living with cancer is a challenging journey that requires strength and courage. It is a journey that can be filled with both joy and sorrow, and it is a journey that no one should have to go through alone. By connecting with others who have gone through similar experiences and by taking care of your physical and mental health, you can gain strength and hope for the future and live your best life despite the challenges.

No matter what life throws your way, you are capable of facing whatever comes your way and living a life full of purpose and meaning.

CHAPTER FIVE
My Fight against Cancer

When I was diagnosed with cancer in 2019, I was overwhelmed with emotion. I had no idea what to expect, and I was terrified of the journey ahead. I had heard stories of other people's battles with cancer, and I had seen the devastating effects it had on their lives. But I was determined to fight and do whatever it took to beat this disease.

In the months that followed, I underwent a series of treatments, including chemotherapy, immunotherapy, and radiation therapy. I was also prescribed medication to help manage my symptoms. The treatments were difficult and sometimes painful, but I was determined to stay strong and keep fighting. I focused on the positive, remembering that each treatment was a step closer to beating cancer.

Throughout my journey, I was supported by an incredible network of family, friends, and healthcare professionals. They were always there to encourage me and provide me with the emotional and physical support I needed. I also sought out support from other cancer survivors, which was invaluable. Hearing their stories and knowing that I wasn't alone in my fight gave me strength and helped me remain hopeful.

I also made sure to take care of myself mentally and physically. Exercise, healthy eating, and stress management became part of my daily routine. I made sure to take breaks for rest and relaxation and to recharge, and I took some time off work when I needed it. I also made sure to spend quality time with my family and friends, as this provided me with a much-needed emotional boost.

Most importantly, I stayed positive and kept my focus on the future. I made sure to look for the silver linings in every situation and to remember that each day was one step closer to beating cancer. Throughout my journey, I kept my eyes on the prize and never gave up.

Eventually, I received the news that I was cancer-free. It was a huge relief, and I felt a great sense of accomplishment. My fight against cancer was one of the toughest things I have ever faced, but I am so thankful that I persevered and won. I have learned a lot from my experience, and I now realize the importance of self-care and positive thinking. I know that I can face any challenge that comes my way and that I am capable of achieving anything I set my mind to.

CHAPTER SIX

My Result, my doubts, my victories

Cancer is a disease that affects millions of people around the world. As a cancer survivor, I have experienced the roller coaster of emotions that come with the diagnosis, treatment, and recovery process. After being diagnosed with cancer, I was faced with a number of difficult decisions. I was faced with the uncertainty of whether I would survive or not, and I had to make a decision about how I was going to fight it.

When I went for my first check-up after being diagnosed with cancer, the doctor told me that I had a good chance of beating it. He said that with the right treatment and dedication, I could beat it. I was filled with hope and optimism, but also a great deal of fear and worry. I had a lot of doubts about my ability to beat this disease. I was scared of the chemotherapy and radiation treatments, and I was worried about what the outcome would be.

Fortunately, after months of intense treatment, I was able to beat the cancer. My result was that I was cancer free. It was a huge victory and a huge relief. I was filled with a deep sense of joy and satisfaction that I had overcome such a difficult disease.

However, my journey with cancer was not over yet. Even after the cancer was gone, I still had to deal with the emotional and physical scars that came with it. I was left with a great deal of doubt and insecurity. I was constantly worried that the cancer would come back. I was scared to death of going through the same treatments and facing the same outcome.

But I was determined to stay strong and not let the doubts take over. I was determined to keep fighting and to keep believing in myself and in my ability to beat the disease. I made a commitment to myself that I would never give up.

Throughout my journey, I have learned many lessons. I have learned that there is no such thing as a guarantee when it comes to beating cancer. I have also learned that it is important to be open to new treatments and to have a positive attitude. It is also important to have a strong support system, both family and friends, who can help you through the tough times.

My experience with cancer has been a long and difficult journey. But despite the doubts and fears, I am proud to say that I am now a cancer survivor. I have had to fight hard and stay strong, but I have also been able to celebrate my victories. I am grateful for the medical professionals who have helped me on this journey and for the support of my family and friends. I am also thankful for my own strength and determination to keep going and to beat this disease.

Cancer is a challenging and difficult journey, but it is possible to beat it. It takes dedication, strength, and perseverance, but it is possible. I am living proof that cancer can be beaten.

CHAPTER SEVEN

My new life objective is to assist others to be cancer free

For many of us, it can be difficult to live life with a purpose and to set meaningful goals. But one of the most fulfilling things that you can do with your life is to help others. That is why my new life goal is to help others to be cancer free.

Cancer is a devastating disease that affects millions of people around the world. It can be incredibly devastating to the ones who suffer from it, and to their loved ones. Watching someone you love battle cancer can be one of the most difficult experiences of your life. That is why it is so important to do everything that you can to help people who are affected by cancer.

One of the best ways that you can help those affected by cancer is to provide emotional support. Whether it is by listening to their stories and offering words of encouragement, or simply being a friend who is there when they need you, it can make a huge difference. It is also important to provide physical support. This could be anything from helping with errands or providing transportation to treatment centers.

In addition to providing emotional and physical support, it is also important to help people affected by cancer with their financial needs. Many people who suffer from cancer struggle to pay for their medical treatment and other expenses that come with the disease. By donating money or offering to help with fundraising, you can make a big difference in someone's life.

Another way to help those affected by cancer is to raise awareness. We can all do our part to spread the word about the importance of early detection and prevention. By educating yourself and those around you about the signs and symptoms of cancer, you could potentially save a life.

Finally, one of the best ways to help those affected by cancer is to get involved with cancer research. Volunteering at a cancer research center or donating to a cancer research foundation can make a huge difference. The more money that is raised for cancer research, the closer we get to finding a cure.

My goal is to help those affected by cancer, and I am committed to doing whatever I can to make a difference. I know that it won't be easy, but I am determined to do my part and I am confident that together, we can make a difference.

My hope is that one day, cancer will no longer be a life sentence. My dream is that everyone affected by cancer will have the opportunity to live a long, healthy life. This is my goal and I am committed to doing whatever it takes to make it happen.

CHAPTER EIGHT

What Causes Cancer?

1. Smoking: Smoking is the leading cause of cancer and is linked to various forms of cancer, including lung, bladder, and pancreatic cancer.

2. Excessive Alcohol Consumption: Drinking too much alcohol is linked to an increased risk of several types of cancer, including mouth, throat, liver, and breast cancer.

3. Obesity: Being overweight or obese increases the risk of several types of cancer, including breast, colorectal, and endometrial cancer.

4. Poor Diet: Eating a diet high in red and processed meats, as well as high in refined

carbohydrates and low in fruits and vegetables, can increase the risk of certain types of cancer.

5. Sun Exposure: Prolonged exposure to UV radiation from the sun can increase the risk of skin cancer.

6. Infection: Certain viruses and bacteria, such as the human papillomavirus (HPV) and Helicobacter pylori, can increase the risk of certain types of cancer.

7. Radiation: Exposure to radiation, such as that from X-rays or other medical procedures, can increase the risk of cancer.

8. Environmental Toxins: Exposure to certain environmental toxins, such as asbestos and benzene, can increase the risk of cancer.

9. Family History: Having a family history of certain cancers can increase the risk of developing them.

10. Hormone Therapy: Long-term use of certain hormone therapies, such as those used to treat prostate cancer, can increase the risk of certain cancers.

11. Genetic Factors: Certain genetic mutations can increase the risk of certain cancers.

12. Smoking During Pregnancy: Smoking during pregnancy can increase the risk of certain types of cancer in children.

13. Age: The risk of developing some types of cancer increases with age.

14. Gender: Men are at higher risk of developing certain types of cancer, such as prostate and lung cancer.

15. Race: African-Americans are at higher risk of developing certain types of cancer, such as colorectal, prostate, and breast cancer.

16. Exposure to Air Pollution: Exposure to air pollution, such as car exhaust, can increase the risk of certain types of cancer.

17. Exposure to Pesticides: Exposure to certain pesticides, such as organochlorines, can increase the risk of certain types of cancer.

18. Exposure to Radiation in the Workplace: People who work in certain industries, such as nuclear power plants or medical diagnostics,

can be exposed to increased levels of radiation, which can increase the risk of certain cancers.

19. Exposure to Industrial Chemicals: Exposure to certain industrial chemicals, such as benzene and vinyl chloride, can increase the risk of certain types of cancer.

20. Exposure to Radiation From Mobile Phones: Some studies have suggested that long-term use of mobile phones may increase the risk of certain types of cancer.

CHAPTER NINE

Cancer Diets

10 Cancer Diets and how they're prepared

1. Roasted Chicken with Asparagus and Tomatoes - Prep time: 30 minutes

Ingredients:

2 skinless, boneless chicken breasts,

2 tablespoons olive oil,

1/2 teaspoon garlic powder,

1/2 teaspoon dried oregano,

1/2 teaspoon salt,

1/4 teaspoon freshly ground pepper,

2 cups asparagus spears,

trimmed, 1 pint cherry tomatoes, halved,

2 tablespoons freshly chopped parsley

2. Baked Salmon with Garlic and Herbs - Prep time: 20 minutes

Ingredients:

4 skinless salmon fillets,

2 tablespoons olive oil,

1 teaspoon garlic powder,

1 teaspoon dried oregano,

1 teaspoon freshly chopped parsley,

1/2 teaspoon salt,

1/4 teaspoon freshly ground black pepper

3. Spinach and Feta Quiche - Prep time: 30 minutes

Ingredients:

1 9-inch unbaked pie crust,

2 tablespoons olive oil,

1/2 onion, diced,

2 cloves garlic, minced,

1 10-ounce package frozen spinach, thawed and squeezed dry,

3 eggs,

1/2 cup grated Parmesan cheese,

1/2 cup crumbled feta cheese,

1 teaspoon dried oregano,

1/2 teaspoon freshly ground black pepper

4. Lentil Soup - Prep time: 30 minutes

Ingredients:

2 tablespoons olive oil,

1 onion, diced,

4 cloves garlic, minced,

2 cups green lentils, rinsed,

8 cups vegetable broth,

1/2 teaspoon cumin,

1/2 teaspoon smoked paprika,

1/2 teaspoon freshly ground pepper,

1 bay leaf,

1/4 cup freshly chopped parsley

5. Kale and Quinoa Salad - Prep time: 15 minutes

Ingredients:

1 cup quinoa, cooked,

2 cups kale, chopped,

1/2 cup sun-dried tomatoes,

1/4 cup slivered almonds,

2 tablespoons olive oil,

1 tablespoon lemon juice,

1/2 teaspoon garlic powder,

1/2 teaspoon dried oregano,

1/4 teaspoon freshly ground black pepper

6. Baked Sweet Potato Fries - Prep time: 25 minutes

Ingredients:

4 large sweet potatoes,

peeled and cut into strips,

2 tablespoons olive oil,

1/2 teaspoon garlic powder,

1/2 teaspoon dried oregano,

1/2 teaspoon smoked paprika,

1/2 teaspoon salt,

1/4 teaspoon freshly ground black pepper

7. Broccoli and Cauliflower Fritters - Prep time: 20 minutes

Ingredients: 1 head broccoli, cut into florets,

1 head cauliflower, cut into florets,

2 eggs, lightly beaten,

1/2 cup all-purpose flour,

1/2 teaspoon garlic powder,

1/2 teaspoon dried oregano,

1/2 teaspoon salt,

1/4 teaspoon freshly ground black pepper,

2 tablespoons olive oil

8. Roasted Brussels Sprouts - Prep time: 20 minutes

Ingredients:

1 pound Brussels sprouts, trimmed and halved,

2 tablespoons olive oil,

1/2 teaspoon garlic powder,

1/2 teaspoon dried oregano,

1/2 teaspoon salt,

1/4 teaspoon freshly ground black pepper

9. Grilled Vegetable Stuffed Portobello Mushrooms - Prep time: 25 minutes

Ingredients:

4 large portobello mushrooms, stems removed,

2 tablespoons olive oil,

1/2 onion, diced,

2 cloves garlic, minced,

1/2 red bell pepper, diced,

1/2 yellow bell pepper, diced,

1/2 teaspoon dried oregano,

1/2 teaspoon smoked paprika,

1/2 teaspoon salt,

1/4 teaspoon freshly ground black pepper

10. Zucchini Noodles with Pesto - Prep time: 10 minutes

Ingredients:

4 zucchini, spiralized,

2 tablespoons olive oil,

2 cloves garlic, minced,

1/2 cup freshly chopped basil,

1/4 cup grated Parmesan cheese,

2 tablespoons pine nuts,

2 tablespoons lemon juice,

1/2 teaspoon salt,

1/4 teaspoon freshly ground black pepper

Bonus: Our free cancer Prevention Secret

100 Secrets on how to Prevent Cancer

1. Exercise regularly: Exercise helps to reduce the risk of several types of cancer by improving overall health, maintaining a healthy weight, and reducing inflammation.

2. Eat a healthy diet: Eating a diet rich in a variety of vegetables, fruits, and whole grains can help to reduce the risk of cancer. Avoiding processed and red meats can also help reduce your risk.

3. Avoid tobacco: Using any type of tobacco is linked to an increased risk of many types of cancer. Avoiding it altogether is the best way to reduce your risk.

4. Get vaccinated: Vaccinating against certain viruses, such as HPV and hepatitis B, can help to reduce the risk of some cancers.

5. Protect your skin: Wearing sunscreen and protective clothing can help to reduce the risk of skin cancer.

6. Limit alcohol: Limiting the amount of alcohol you consume has been linked to a lower risk of certain types of cancer.

7. Avoid environmental pollutants: Exposure to pollutants, such as radon, asbestos, and other chemicals, can increase the risk of cancer.

8. Get screened: Regular screenings can help to detect cancer early and improve the chances of successful treatment.

9. Maintain a healthy weight: Being overweight or obese can increase the risk of certain types of cancer.

10. Eat foods rich in antioxidants: Eating foods that are rich in antioxidants, such as berries and dark leafy greens, can help to reduce the risk of cancer.

11. Avoid exposure to radiation: Exposure to radiation can increase the risk of certain types of cancer.

12. Limit sugar intake: Eating too much sugar can increase the risk of certain types of cancer.

13. Avoid processed foods: Processed foods can contain additives that can increase the risk of cancer.

14. Avoid risky behaviors: Risky behaviors, such as sharing needles, can increase the risk of certain types of cancer.

15. Get enough sleep: Not getting enough sleep can increase the risk of certain types of cancer.

16. Avoid grilled and barbecued meats: Eating grilled and barbecued meats can increase the risk of certain types of cancer.

17. Limit exposure to pesticides: Pesticides can contain chemicals that can increase the risk of certain types of cancer.

18. Choose organic foods: Choosing organic foods can reduce your exposure to pesticides and other chemicals that can increase the risk of cancer.

19. Eat more garlic: Eating garlic can help to reduce the risk of certain types of cancer.

20. Drink green tea: Drinking green tea can help to reduce the risk of certain types of cancer.

21. Limit red meat intake: Eating too much red meat has been linked to an increased risk of certain types of cancer.

22. Eat more cruciferous vegetables: Cruciferous vegetables, such as broccoli and cabbage, can help to reduce the risk of certain types of cancer.

23. Avoid hormone replacement therapy: Long-term use of hormone replacement

therapy has been linked to an increased risk of certain types of cancer.

24. Avoid artificial sweeteners: Artificial sweeteners can contain chemicals that can increase the risk of certain types of cancer.

25. Limit your exposure to sunlight: Too much exposure to sunlight can increase the risk of skin cancer.

26. Avoid BPA: BPA, a chemical found in plastic, can increase the risk of certain types of cancer.

27. Avoid trans fats: Trans fats, found in processed and fried foods, can increase the risk of certain types of cancer.

28. Avoid microwaving food in plastic containers: Microwaving food in plastic containers can increase the risk of certain types of cancer due to leaching of chemicals.

29. Eat more fish: Eating more fish can help to reduce the risk of certain types of cancer.

30. Limit your consumption of processed meats: Eating too much processed meat, such

as bacon and hot dogs, can increase the risk of certain types of cancer.

31. Avoid air pollution: Exposure to air pollution can increase the risk of certain types of cancer.

32. Limit your exposure to household chemicals: Household chemicals, such as bleach and detergents, can increase the risk of certain types of cancer.

33. Eat more fiber: Eating more fiber can help to reduce the risk of certain types of cancer.

34. Avoid Bovine Growth Hormone (rBGH): Milk and other dairy products that have been treated with Bovine Growth Hormone can increase the risk of certain types of cancer.

35. Avoid saturated fat: Eating too much saturated fat can increase the risk of certain types of cancer.

36. Eat more soy: Eating more soy can help to reduce the risk of certain types of cancer.

37. Avoid refined carbohydrates: Eating too many refined carbohydrates, such as white

bread and pasta, can increase the risk of certain types of cancer.

38. Limit your consumption of deli meats: Eating too many deli meats, such as salami and ham, can increase the risk of certain types of cancer.

39. Drink filtered water: Drinking filtered water can reduce your exposure to pollutants that can increase the risk of certain types of cancer.

40. Avoid canned foods: Canned foods can contain chemicals that can increase the risk of certain types of cancer.

41. Avoid charred foods: Eating charred foods can increase the risk of certain types of cancer.

42. Avoid hydrogenated oils: Eating too much hydrogenated oils, such as margarine and shortening, can increase the risk of certain types of cancer.

43. Get tested for HIV: HIV can increase the risk of certain types of cancer.

44. Limit your exposure to x-rays: Too much exposure to x-rays can increase the risk of certain types of cancer.

45. Avoid canned beverages: Canned beverages can contain chemicals that can increase the risk of certain types of cancer.

46. Avoid artificial food dyes: Eating too many artificial food dyes can increase the risk of certain types of cancer.

47. Avoid nitrate-rich foods: Eating too much nitrate-rich foods, such as cured meats and

lunch meats, can increase the risk of certain types of cancer.

48. Limit your exposure to household cleaners: Household cleaners can contain chemicals that can increase the risk of certain types of cancer.

49. Avoid artificial sweeteners: Artificial sweeteners can contain chemicals that can increase the risk of certain types of cancer.

50. Avoid chemical-based pesticides: Chemical-based pesticides can contain chemicals that can increase the risk of certain types of cancer.

51. Drink more water: Drinking more water can help to reduce the risk of certain types of cancer.

52. Eat more fruits and vegetables: Eating more fruits and vegetables can help to reduce the risk of certain types of cancer.

53. Avoid hormone therapy: Long-term use of hormone therapy can increase the risk of certain types of cancer.

54. Avoid sugary drinks: Drinking sugary drinks, such as soda and energy drinks, can increase the risk of certain types of cancer.

55. Avoid charred and grilled foods: Eating charred and grilled foods, such as barbecued meats, can increase the risk of certain types of cancer.

56. Avoid chemical-based sunscreens: Chemical-based sunscreens can contain chemicals that can increase the risk of certain types of cancer.

57. Avoid processed vegetable oils: Eating too much processed vegetable oils, such as canola and soybean oil, can increase the risk of certain types of cancer.

58. Avoid canned soups: Canned soups can contain chemicals that can increase the risk of certain types of cancer.

59. Eat more nuts and seeds: Eating more nuts and seeds can help to reduce the risk of certain types of cancer.

60. Avoid second-hand smoke: Second-hand smoke can increase the risk of certain types of cancer.

61. Limit your alcohol consumption: Drinking too much alcohol can increase the risk of certain types of cancer.

62. Avoid fried foods: Eating too many fried foods can increase the risk of certain types of cancer.

63. Avoid deli meats: Eating too many deli meats, such as salami and ham, can increase the risk of certain types of cancer.

64. Avoid refined sugars: Eating too much refined sugar can increase the risk of certain types of cancer.

65. Avoid charred and blackened foods: Eating charred and blackened foods, such as barbecued meats, can increase the risk of certain types of cancer.

66. Avoid canned fruits and vegetables: Canned fruits and vegetables can contain chemicals that can increase the risk of certain types of cancer.

67. Avoid nitrate-rich processed meats: Eating too many processed meats, such as bacon and hot dogs, can increase the risk of certain types of cancer.

68. Avoid microwaving food in plastic containers: Microwaving food in plastic containers can increase the risk of certain types of cancer due to leaching of chemicals.

69. Avoid canned fish: Canned fish can contain chemicals that can increase the risk of certain types of cancer.

70. Avoid polyunsaturated fats: Eating too much polyunsaturated fats, such as margarine and shortening, can increase the risk of certain types of cancer.

71. Avoid artificial coloring: Eating too many artificial colors can increase the risk of certain types of cancer.

72. Avoid canned soups and sauces: Canned soups and sauces can contain chemicals that can increase the risk of certain types of cancer.

73. Avoid non-stick cookware: Non-stick cookware can contain chemicals that can increase the risk of certain types of cancer.

74. Avoid microwaving food in Styrofoam containers: Microwaving food in Styrofoam containers can increase the risk of certain types of cancer due to leaching of chemicals.

75. Limit your exposure to environmental pollutants: Exposure to environmental pollutants, such as radon, asbestos, and other chemicals, can increase the risk of cancer.

76. Avoid canned juices: Canned juices can contain chemicals that can increase the risk of certain types of cancer.

77. Drink less soda: Drinking too much soda can increase the risk of certain types of cancer.

78. Avoid processed grains: Eating too many processed grains, such as white bread and pasta, can increase the risk of certain types of cancer.

79. Eat more fresh fruits and vegetables: Eating more fresh fruits and vegetables can help to reduce the risk of certain types of cancer.

80. Avoid chemical-based cleaning products: Chemical-based cleaning products can contain chemicals that can increase the risk of certain types of cancer.

81. Avoid foods containing artificial preservatives: Eating too many foods containing artificial preservatives can increase the risk of certain types of cancer.

82. Avoid grilled and barbecued meats: Eating grilled and barbecued meats can increase the risk of certain types of cancer.

83. Avoid fried foods: Eating too many fried foods can increase the risk of certain types of cancer.

84. Avoid processed meats: Eating too many processed meats, such as bacon and hot dogs, can increase the risk of certain types of cancer.

85. Avoid canned beans and legumes: Canned beans and legumes can contain chemicals that can increase the risk of certain types of cancer.

86. Avoid non-organic dairy products: Non-organic dairy products can contain hormones

and antibiotics that can increase the risk of certain types of cancer.

87. Avoid canned tomatoes: Canned tomatoes can contain chemicals that can increase the risk of certain types of cancer.

88. Avoid canned fish: Canned fish can contain chemicals that can increase the risk of certain types of cancer.

89. Avoid foods containing high levels of sodium: Eating too many foods containing high levels of sodium can increase the risk of certain types of cancer.

90. Avoid canned soups: Canned soups can contain chemicals that can increase the risk of certain types of cancer.

91. Avoid white flour: Eating too much white flour can increase the risk of certain types of cancer.

92. Avoid canned fruits: Canned fruits can contain chemicals that can increase the risk of certain types of cancer.

93. Avoid processed snacks: Eating too many processed snacks, such as chips and crackers, can increase the risk of certain types of cancer.

94. Avoid canned vegetables: Canned vegetables can contain chemicals that can increase the risk of certain types of cancer.

95. Avoid chemical-based fertilizers: Chemical-based fertilizers can contain chemicals that can increase the risk of certain types of cancer.

96. Avoid chemical-based insecticides: Chemical-based insecticides can contain

chemicals that can increase the risk of certain types of cancer.

97. Limit your exposure to artificial light: Too much exposure to artificial light, such as fluorescent lights, can increase the risk of certain types of cancer.

98. Avoid fatty meats: Eating too much fatty meats, such as bacon and hot dogs, can increase the risk of certain types of cancer.

99. Avoid artificial sweeteners: Artificial sweeteners can contain chemicals that can increase the risk of certain types of cancer.

100. Avoid canned beverages: Canned beverages can contain chemicals that can increase the risk of certain types of cancer.

Conclusion

Cancer is a devastating disease that has taken too many lives and left too many families and friends devastated. But it is also a reminder of the strength of the human spirit and how we can come together to fight such a devastating illness. The progress in treatments and the strides made in research and clinical trials give us hope that one day we will have a cure for this dreadful disease. We must continue to support those who are fighting cancer and never give up hope. We must remember those who have lost their battle with cancer and the loved ones they left behind. We must continue to be a light of hope in the darkness and fight together for a world free of cancer.

www.ingramcontent.com/pod-product-compliance
Lightning Source LLC
LaVergne TN
LVHW052050160826
845678LV00015B/3148

* 9 7 9 8 3 7 1 1 9 0 3 8 3 *